Mind Matters

A resource bank on

SELF-ESTEEM

"What if..........?"   Marilyn Harvey

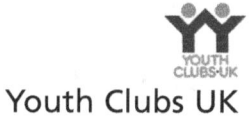
Youth Clubs UK

Acknowledgements

We would like to thank

Pauline Taylor for managing the Mind Matters project

Gail Russell and Jane Saunders for contributing to the writing process

Tobin Florio for designing the front cover

Geraldine Ryan for design and typesetting

Martha Florio for proof-reading

Cheshire and Wirral Federation of Youth Clubs for a summary of their Young Men's Project Phase Two

The Department of Health who contributed funds for the development of the Mind Matters project

And lastly, we would like to thank our young models who posed for the photographs

Published by Youth Clubs UK 2000 ©

2nd Floor, Kirby House
Kirby Street
London EC1N 8TS
Telephone: 020 7 242 4045
Fax: 020 7 242 4125
E-mail: youthclubs.uk@ukonline.co.uk
Website: http://www.youthclubs.org.uk/main.htm

Reg. Charity No. 306066

ISBN O 907095 09 7

INTRODUCTION

About

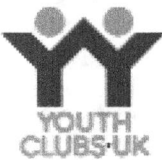 Youth Clubs UK, a national registered charity, promotes opportunities for young people to develop skills and interests which will help them to become fulfilled adults and effective citizens.

It is the largest non-uniformed youth organization in the United Kingdom, supporting a network that reaches more than 700,000 young people in clubs and projects and including about 45,000 youth workers with over 30,000 volunteers.

Youth Clubs UK initiates a wide range of projects - for example art, drama, dance, health education, action to improve the environment, community work and international exchanges.

The organization also works with particular disadvantaged groups such as homeless young people or those involved with car crime, drugs, alcohol or solvents.

The key aim of our work is to give young people, whatever their starting point, the skills and information they need to make constructive decisions and to plan and manage their own activities and projects.

About the Author

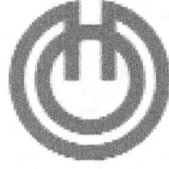 Marilyn Harvey is a qualified nurse and social worker who has been involved in the field of mental health since 1980. Marilyn has extensive experience working with adults and young people who have had short and long term mental health problems.

More recently she has been involved in developing a variety of mental health promotion projects and courses. She is the author of a number of publications related to health and social care issues and has been involved in developing youth work projects for 18 years.

SELF-ESTEEM

Contents

Introduction
Part One

About Mind Matters

Mental health is not something that people generally talk about or even understand very well. We seem to be much better at knowing when our physical health and bodies are well or ill. You could say mental health is about feeling good about oneself, being aware of what you are like and respecting oneself so that you can take control of your own life and make your own decisions.

Youth Clubs UK strongly supports the view that good mental health is more than the absence of mental illness. One way that the organization is promoting this idea is by launching a series of 5 resource banks similar to this one. Each one will enable trainers, youth workers and teachers to explore a range of issues related to mental health issues, with groups of young people. The aim is to get young people thinking about how they can look after their own mental health and support their friends and others when they are experiencing some kind of trauma and/or distress.

Why have a resource bank on self-esteem?

The term 'self-esteem' is a relatively modern one as a day-to-day word. In the past it was more frequently used amongst professional doctors, psychologists, social workers and others in the educational and mental health field. During recent years however it is a word that is often used by lay people and can be read about in a variety of magazines, books and so on.

During recent years those in the mental health field have come to realize that the way individuals feel about themselves can help or hinder both their physical, mental, spiritual and emotional health. Feelings associated with high or low self-esteem can also influence and sometimes govern the way individuals behave both in private and in public.

It is therefore important that those who work alongside young people enable them to explore how their self-esteem is developed, and what factors can influence the way they feel about themselves and behave towards others. It is also of equal importance that young people are given opportunities to learn some of the skills that may help an individual to improve their self-esteem. For example learning how to resist peer pressure to be involved in activities that make a young person feel bad about themselves afterwards are important skills that will help young people to feel more positive and assertive. Learning how to give compliments, and becoming more aware of how as an individual one puts others down, are two examples of the ways that young people can develop important and essential life skills.

The three quotes below all highlight young people with different levels of self-esteem:

"I am 14 years old and I suffer really badly with spots. My mum took me to the doctor who gave me some cream but the spots are still there. I know they look really awful and I hate going to school in case anyone makes fun of me. A boy asked me out last week and I said no because I know I will get lots of spots and he will dump me. Sometimes I feel so miserable about the way I look that I just cry myself to sleep and hope I die."

"At school one of the teachers keeps picking on me all of the time. I don't know what I have done to make her hate me but she only ever picks on me and not my friends. If there is any trouble in the class I always get blamed for it even if I am sitting somewhere else. I am the only one who gets detention from her and it is really upsetting me. I want to ask her what I have done wrong but I am scared that she will just shout at me... I just don't know what to do about it."

"I just want to be allowed to go out like a normal teenager but my mum wouldn't let me. I have got some learning disabilities and go to a special school. My mum says I am not like other boys of 16 and it's better I don't go out and get attached to any girls because that will only upset me when they find out what I am really like. Sometimes I feel so lonely, hopeless and odd but I don't feel I can do anything about it really."

These examples show different reasons why young people might be experiencing a low self-esteem. They have two things in common. In all three situations the young people described feel bad inside themselves, whilst also feeling that they are powerless to do anything about their circumstances.

Many feel at present that young people experience problems dealing with their inner feelings because they lack understanding of the normality of them and/or they worry that they might be laughed at or perceived as odd if they were to speak about them.

Others argue that the main reason that young people often feel isolated, rejected, useless and undervalued, whatever their circumstances, is because their friends and other adults around them do not know what to say and how to support them.

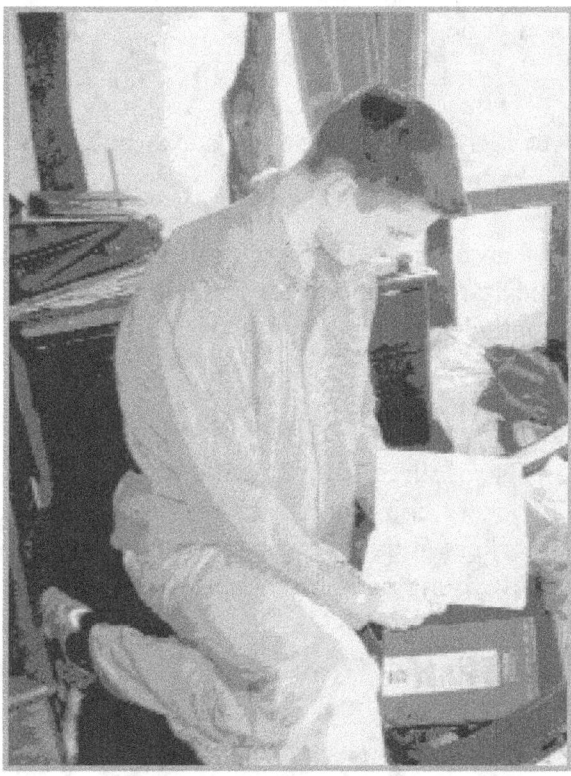

The aim of this resource bank is to provide activities that will enable you to help young people explore some of the feelings and issues that are associated with different levels of self-esteem and ways they might help themselves feel better about who they are.

Because mental health issues are such an integral part of our society, it is important that young people explore the issues concerned with self-esteem, both in terms of their own health and the part they play in supporting or stigmatising others in society.

What does this resource bank include?

— Guidelines on facilitating activities about self-esteem with young people,

— information about the nature of self-esteem and how it impacts on young people,

— photocopiable learning activities that workers can use or adapt to increase young people's awareness and understanding about self-esteem,

— an outline of a Peer Health Education project that used drama to facilitate opportunities for young to explore issues that affect their mental well-being.

Who is this resource bank for?

This resource bank has been designed for voluntary and paid youth workers, community workers, teachers, health promotion staff, social workers and other professionals who want to work in partnership with young people to explore a range of mental health issues.

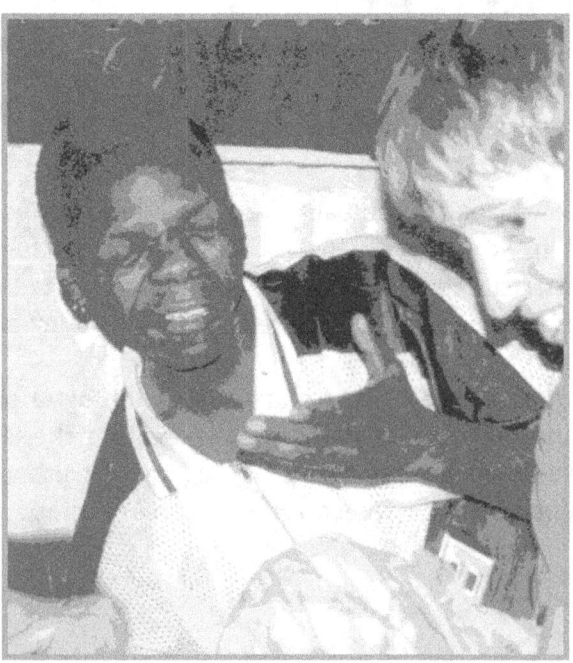

The person using this manual will need to have some understanding of working with young people exploring subjects and issues that impinge on their day-to-day life. It is also important that the worker co-ordinating the project has experience of working with young people in groups, and has access to health promotion or other specialist agencies for advice and support about any issues that might be raised in relation to self-esteem.

How can this resource bank be used?

All the activities in this publication have been set out for use with young people who meet together for an agreed learning programme. This could take place in various youth work settings.

Some workers may choose to use the activities on one-day courses or weekly sessions. Others might use the activities during a residential course. The setting might be a formal or an informal one but it is recommended that the following issues are carefully considered before embarking on any of the activities.

Size of group:

It is important that the group size is small enough to allow every participant to contribute, but not so small that a young person might feel put on the spot. Around 6-8 young people is a good size for a discussion group. If by necessity you work with a much larger group, for example a class of 20, it's especially important that the activities are done in small groups with large group input being kept to a minimum.

The setting:

Create a safe environment for the young people to share with each other. Choose a comfortable room which is private, where you are not likely to be disturbed. Chairs in a circle can create a more intimate feel and everyone can see or hear what everyone else is doing. Young people also like to sit on the floor when having a group discussion.

Provision of materials:

Check you have all the materials required e.g. paper, pens, blu-tac, sufficient photocopies of the exercises etc. If using audio-visual equipment, check it is working before you start.

Negotiating boundaries:

Clarity about timing is important for people to feel safe. Remember to let people know when something is to begin and end and when there will be breaks. If you ask participants to do an exercise, be precise about how long they will have to complete it and let them know what will happen afterwards e.g. "After you have finished I will ask your group to feedback to everyone else 3 important points you discussed." If you are going to change these agreements it is important to discuss it with the group.

Ground Rules:

The group will need to establish a few ground rules in order to feel secure and respected. Confidentiality and respect for each other's viewpoint is essential. Participants should also be reassured that the activities will not result in them having to share any personal stories about their own self-esteem problems, but it's up to them if they wish to share personal information during any discussions. Rules may also include; only one person speaking at a time, agreements about smoking and so on. It is essential to discuss a ground rule about dropping out of the activity, in the event that a participant finds it stressful due to some kind of difficult situation going on in their own life.

Respect for differences:

It is important to foster a climate in which any differences in a group such as class, race, culture, sexuality or disability are seen as positive. Participants should be encouraged to respect differences rather than see their own views as the right ones.

Backup support:

Sometimes it is difficult to predict how groups are going to react to exploring mental issues like self-esteem. In many incidences the activities are likely to go down well and the young people will gain from being involved and will leave the session in a positive and questioning frame of mind. There may be occasions though when a participant bumps into one of their stressful experiences and feels distressed as a result of the activities. It is therefore important that somebody is available who can respond to this kind of situation at the end of a session. It is also helpful to have the names and addresses of your local young people's support agencies in the event that a participant would like more help for themselves after having explored some issues about young people and self-esteem.

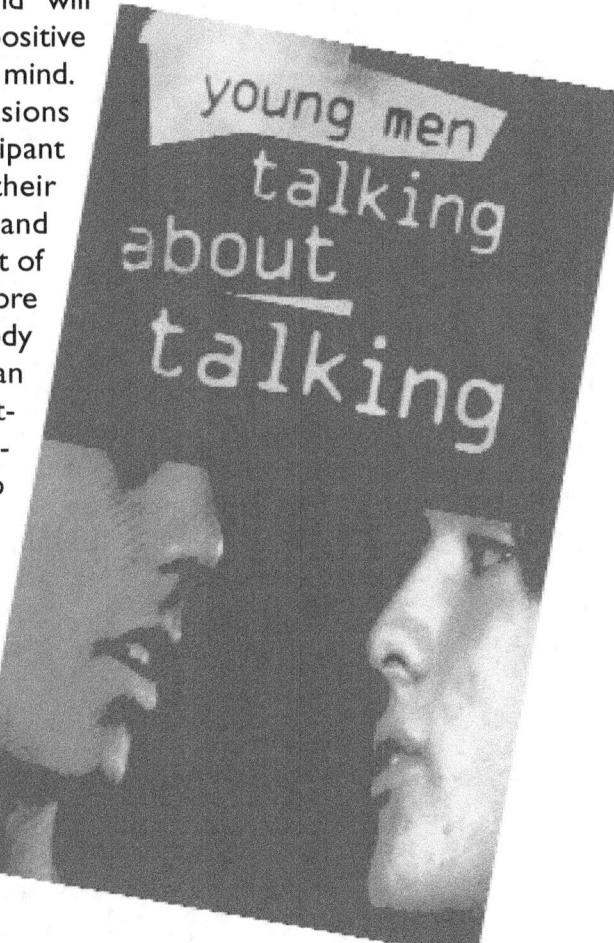

It is important to ask the group if they have other things they want to discuss and agree in order to help them feel they can participate fully in the activities.

Things to remember when facilitating activities

Introductions

Warm-ups, or icebreakers as they are also known, are considered to be important at the start of group activities because participants become actively involved with each other from the outset. This is of basic importance if the activities are of a participatory nature.

Warm-ups help the individuals to start seeing themselves as a group. A cautionary note needs to be made about the use of warm-ups. It is vital that the course facilitator chooses warm-ups which are appropriate for the individuals in the group at that time. The informal nature of warm-ups and their potential for a certain degree of self-revelation can mean that, if used inappropriately, they can be very threatening to some participants. The outcome is that they can make people feel more uncomfortable rather than more comfortable and so defeat their purpose. Here are some examples of warm-ups that could be used.

The name game

starts with the course facilitator who says "my name is ...." It then moves to the person on the facilitator's left (or right) who says "My name is ...., and this (the course facilitator) is ...." and so on, until the tenth person, for example, has to remember ten names (including his/her own!) Generally speaking, this game can be played successfully with up to 15 course participants.

Another name game

Aim

Getting to know people's names and something about them

This exercise is excellent for small groups. It can be used for up to twenty participants, but once the numbers get above twelve, it may be better to divide into two or more small groups, rather than have so many names to listen to at once.

You'll need

Large sheets of paper/flipchart
Felt-tip/marker pens

What to do

Ask the participants to sit in a circle either on chairs or on the floor with the pens and paper in the centre of the circle, then invite each participant to go to the centre in turn and write their name using a coloured pen on the paper.

As they do so, ask them to share one or two sentences about their names, for example, why they were given that name, if they like their names or not, or something that gives a picture that helps the group remember who they are.

You may like to invite people to do this in any order which gives the shy ones time to pluck up courage and think of something to say. It usually means that most people have learnt the names by the end of the exercise.

Variation

Ask participants to select an article of clothing that they like and as well as sharing their names, they might want to say something about the clothing. An illustration of this might be "I'm wearing this jumper because it is very colourful and warm and was given to me for Christmas by my boyfriend."

Conversation in twos/Conversation in fours

Divide people into pairs and each person is asked to tell their partner for, say, 3 minutes, a little about themselves (what they share is for them to choose). The partner is asked to listen attentively and sometimes put in comments to reflect what is being said. They are asked, however, not to add their own observations/anecdotes/advice. The roles are then reversed.

The course facilitator can, if appropriate, provide starting sentences for this, like:

"The things that make me happy are.........."
"What I really want to get from this course is.........."

The pairs are then asked to join with another pair and are asked to introduce their partner, sharing briefly some of the information they learned. Each of the four players takes a turn.

The course facilitator needs to stress that anything which could be deemed as confidential should not be shared in this activity.

Finishing activities

Ending games, as they are also known, are considered to be important at the end of group activities because participants can actively wind down and leave on a positive note. Here are some examples that could be used.

"Today I........"

Ask the participants, in turn, to say one thing about the session.

Pairs

Pair up with the person next to you and tell each other how you feel, then do the same again with the person on your other side.

Evaluation sheets

Draw up a simple evaluation sheet so that members of the group can leave behind a note of what they feel or think. This may be done by just writing a comment, negative or positive, on a large sheet of paper or answering some questions.

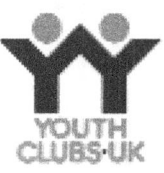

Self-esteem
Part Two

What do we mean by our self-esteem?

"I knew I'd never do very well at school, because that's what every-one always told me. I suppose I didn't disappoint anyone - I just lived up to their expectations."
Karen age 18.

"My mum and dad always told us that if we tried really hard we could be successful at whatever we did, no matter what anyone else said. I think knowing we had that sort of support behind us gave us the confidence to try new things without worrying about how well we might do, or what other people might think."
Andrew age 16.

"I always think everyone looks better than me. I look in the mirror and think how fat and ugly I am, then I don't want to go out and meet people because I know they'll think I'm fat and ugly as well."
Neeta age 15.

"My family don't take any interest in me, so why should I bother. If no one cares about me, maybe I'm just not worth caring about. That's why I take drugs - it makes not caring easier."
Danny age 17.

"I can't remember anyone ever saying anything nice to me when I was little. All I ever wanted was to feel that someone loved me - that's how I ended up pregnant when I was 14. I thought sleeping with boys would make them love me, but it didn't work - they just took what they wanted then went away."
Paige age 17.

"I spent years thinking everyone was better than me, then I got this teacher who made me realize that I was important, and that nobody was better than me. Once I'd convinced myself that she was right I felt much happier, and started doing a lot better at school. What you thought in the past doesn't have to be what you think in the future - it is possible to change if you really want to." Ann age 14.

"I've been in care since I was 2 years old. I've always been looked after properly but no one really loved me. Sometimes I think no-one will ever love me because I just don't deserve it."
Sophie age 13.

What is self-esteem?

Self-esteem can be described as the way we feel and think about ourselves - our feeling of self-worth. From birth onwards a variety of inputs, such as the way we are treated by other people, what they say to us, what we see around us and how we actually feel ourselves help to develop our self-perception. Even as children we start to compare our self-image, or how we see ourselves in reality, with our ideal image, or how we would like other people to see us. If the difference between what we consider to be reality and our ideal image is not too great then we are likely to have a high level of self-esteem. If, however, we perceive the reality as differing widely from the ideal then our level of self-esteem may be considerably lower.

For young people issues relating to self-esteem can be particularly important. Adolescence is a time when many changes take place, both physically and emotionally; young people can be especially sensitive at this time, becoming very critical of themselves. They do not necessarily see themselves as others see them, often thinking they are less attractive and accomplished than their peers. Physical disabilities such as being unable to walk, or being asthmatic, can be magnified at a time when it is important to be like everyone else. Young people with learning difficulties may also feel that being 'different' makes it difficult to feel good about themselves. In some cases, possibly as a result of what is seen through the Media, young people can develop an unrealistic concept of what is 'normal'. They may see pop stars in magazines, sports personalities and other young people on the television, all seeming to be 'perfect'. Failure to comply with this idealised normality may lead to feelings of low self-worth, particularly if peers are also perceived, rightly or wrongly, as being more successful and competent.

Healthy, positive self-esteem is a result of feeling secure and having self-respect, feeling confident enough to deal with life's challenges. It is also concerned with feeling worthy of our own happiness, as well as the respect of others.

Why do people have low self-esteem?

As children our self-image is formed largely by what other people tell us. Everyone has a basic need to receive unconditional positive regard, and most of us receive this from at least one parent, if not from other members of the family. As a child, knowing that you are loved no matter what provides a sound basis for positive self-regard, but for some people this is not the case. Many young people live in dysfunctional families or in environments where they have no family around them at all. In some circumstances it may be that receiving any kind of positive input from others has always been conditional on certain behaviours, therefore it is very difficult to find the confidence to try out new things, or even to develop their own personalities fully, because they fear disapproval.

Some people from an early age encounter more negative input than positive input. In many families children receive far more negative than positive feedback from parents. Parents are quick to chastise children, whereas much behaviour that could receive praise goes unnoticed. If children are constantly told that they are worthless then they come to believe that as being the truth, and will therefore act in accordance with that belief. This can be further perpetuated at school, where because of their low self-esteem they may be low academic achievers, and therefore receive further negative feedback from teachers who perpetuate their belief that they will never 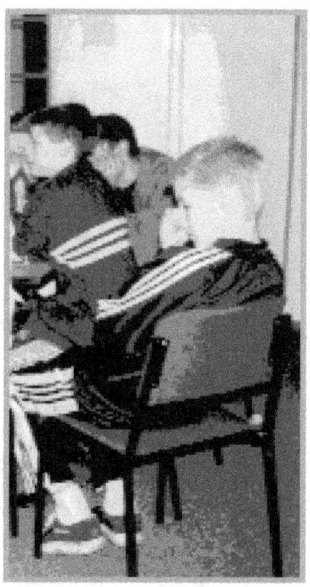 amount to anything. It is important to note that having high self-esteem does not necessarily mean that high academic levels will be attained. What it does mean is that a person is better equipped to do their best and to be happy with the results.

Our environment can cause us to have low self-esteem. Cultural differences and language difficulties for young people such as Asians living in a predominantly European environment can lead to feelings of low self-worth, in some cases perpetuated by the way they are treated by others. Some young people living in care or in foster homes may also feel that they have little to feel good about, and more importantly, that they do not have the power to change their situation. In such instances it can, sometimes, be extremely difficult to alter levels of self-esteem.

How does self-esteem affect us?

If we have a healthy, positive self-esteem it is more likely that we will achieve the goals we set for ourselves in life. We believe that we are capable of reaching our goals, and because of this belief we are more likely to be successful. We are less likely to be influenced by the negativity of others, and may not feel the need to conform to set patterns. If for example young people with a high level of self-esteem were in a situation where drugs or alcohol were being misused, they might have the confidence and strength to say no without worrying too much about not fitting in with their peers.

If on the other hand our self-esteem is low, our success may be hindered by the fact that we do not believe in ourselves. We may feel unable to achieve any goals, therefore have no motivation to set any goals for ourselves. We may also feel unworthy of other people's praise and respect, and because of this will try to devalue others by being negative towards them.

When considering how self-esteem can affect young people it is important to think about conformity. It is often necessary for adolescents to feel that they are the same as their peers - they like the same music, wear the same clothes etc. Although this is a normal part of growing up, young people with low self-esteem may find themselves more susceptible to influence from others around them, particularly those involved in anti-social behaviours. They may feel a greater need for approval, and will therefore strive to do what they feel is expected of them. This can lead them into such behaviour as bullying or being bullied, alcohol and drug abuse and unwanted pregnancies.

If we feel that we are worthless, we will readily believe negative things about ourselves - if, for example a bully tells us we deserve to be beaten up we may believe them. If however we feel good about ourselves we know that we do not deserve to be treated badly, nor do others deserve to be treated badly, therefore we are less likely to become involved in anti-social behaviours.

Can we change the way we feel about ourselves?

Levels of self-esteem are not fixed, although for some people continual negative reinforcement can make it difficult to change. Thinking 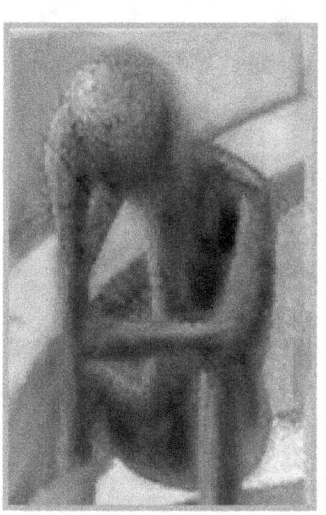 negative thoughts about ourselves can become a habit, often formed in childhood, but it is a habit that can be broken - it is possible to foster a healthy self-esteem. If we think we can do something then we have a good chance of doing it, whereas if we think we can't, we are unlikely to be successful. This indicates that the health of our self-esteem may be dependent on what we think. The power to raise it lies within our own thoughts and what we actually say to ourselves. However, for some people external factors over which they have no control make it very difficult to overcome feelings of low self-worth. Many young people in disadvantaged environments, such as those in care or living on the streets, may feel that they have no control over what happens to them, and that thinking positive thoughts is simply not enough.

How can we raise self-esteem?

One of the most effective ways to change the way we think about our-selves is to change the way we talk to ourselves. Whether we are con-scious of it or not we are constantly telling ourselves how we think or feel. Because of this the way young people communicate with and behave towards each other can either help or hinder self-esteem. Some examples of the sort of things we might say to ourselves are: -

— I feel really good in these clothes.
— This just makes me look fat.
— Everyone gets better marks than I do - I might as well not bother.
— I think I did a good job of that.
— Who cares what I think anyway?
— I can do this if I really try.
— What's the point - I'll never do that in a million years.
— That job is too good for me.

Our minds believe what we tell them, so if we continually tell it we can't do something our actions will bear out those thoughts. We can then become part of a vicious circle, whereby we continually reaffirm our failures, and therefore continue to fail.

As well as improving our own self-esteem we can help to make other people feel good about themselves by taking care about how we talk to them. Some ways that this can be achieved include: -

— Referring to people by name if possible. This will make them feel that you are genuinely interested in them as a person.

— Giving people lots of praise. If you need to criticise, try to do it in a positive way.

— Avoiding being condescending, particularly when offering sympathy. Telling someone that you feel sorry for them may not help them to feel good about themselves, whereas acknowledg-ing their feelings will have a more positive effect.

— Try not to put people down. Everyone benefits from a com-pliment - the giver gains the satisfaction of making someone feel good and the receiver feels respected and appreciated. It is important to be able to accept compliments, and to feel that you deserve to receive them, for example, "you did a really good job there" should be met with a positive reply such as "Thank you for telling me" rather than a negative "No, I didn't".

Rejecting a compliment can make our subconscious believe that the rejection is the truth. If we compare how we feel giving and receiving both compliments and insults we can see that an insult only serves to perpetuate negative feelings which are helpful to no one.

Although we can raise our levels of self-esteem from within, there are many cases where this is not enough, and some external help may be needed. Where young people have no control over their culture, environment or disabilities, we as a society need to think of ways of improving both their circumstances, and they way they are treated. In this way they can at least be given an opportunity to feel good about themselves rather than being made to feel like excluded indviduals.

Who benefits from having positive self-esteem?

The simple answer to this question is that everyone benefits from having positive self-esteem. Individually, our performance and achievement levels will improve if we feel good about and have confidence in ourselves. We are likely to treat other people with more care and respect, and so others may begin to treat us in the same way. The benefits therefore are not only limited to the individual, but can be spread throughout the community.

Encouraging people to raise their level of self-esteem does not mean that everyone will succeed in everything they do and that life will be perfect. What it can mean is that any failures encountered can be turned into a positive learning experience.

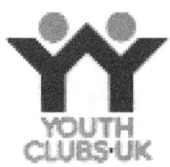

Activities
Part three

SELF-ESTEEM - WHAT SPRINGS TO MIND?

Aim

To get participants thinking about words or phrases that can be associated with positive and negative self-esteem.

You'll need

Large sheets of paper/flipchart
Felt-tip/marker pens
Blu-tac
Dictionary

Time

35 - 45 minutes

What to do

❶ Introduce the session by explaining to the group that they will be looking at 'self-esteem' and words or phrases associated with building both positive and negative 'self-esteem'.

❷ To get people thinking about the word 'self-esteem' you might want to read one or two dictionary definitions or write these on a large sheet of paper/flipchart and have them spread out around the room for people to read before they divide up into groups.

❸ Split the participants up into smaller groups and ask them to discuss words or phrases that come to their mind when they think about high or low self-esteem. Ask them to list the words or phrases on a large sheet of paper. Allow 10 to 15 minutes for this activity. Then bring the participants back into a large group.

❹ Write the words SELF-ESTEEM at the top of the large sheet of paper/flipchart and invite small groups, in turn, to share one idea that they discussed in their small groups. Continue until all the small groups have shared their ideas. (See page 35 for examples of different words or phrases).

ACTIVITY ONE

SELF-ESTEEM - WHAT SPRINGS TO MIND?

Discussion

You may want to broaden the discussion by asking participants to comment on the words or phrases that have been listed on the large sheets of paper/flipchart.

Can they think of any TV actors who come across as having a very low or high self-esteem?

If they can, can they pinpoint any influences that may have led to this?

Variations

— You could ask participants to draw pictures to illustrate the words or phrases already given on page 35 rather than thinking up their own words.

— You could ask participants to put their flipchart paper on the floor or walls and walk around and read each other's ideas rather than asking the small groups to give verbal feedback.

ENDING POINTS

It is important to emphasize that everyone is different and what may raise one person's self-esteem may lower another person's, and vice versa.

ACTIVITY ONE

SELF-ESTEEM - WHAT SPRINGS TO MIND?

nobody loves me

he's found someone else

I always do the best I can

I'm a nice person

I'm useless

I feel good about myself

I can't do anything right

self-worth

good self-image

I like myself

it's all my fault

positive attitude

I did well today

I'm frightened

ACTIVITY ONE

WHAT DO I DO TO MAKE PEOPLE FEEL GOOD OR BAD ABOUT THEMSELVES?

Aim

To get participants thinking about how they can affect other young people's self-esteem.

You'll need

Large sheets of paper/flipchart
Felt-tip/marker pens
Photocopies of 'examples of actions that can raise or lower self-esteem'
(see page 39)

Time

30 - 45 minutes

What to do

❶ Introduce the session by explaining to the group that they will be looking at how they can make other people feel good or bad about themselves.

❷ Split the participants up into groups of 4 and give each group a large sheet of paper and some felt tip/marker pens.

❸ Ask them to write a list of actions that they think might raise or lower someone's self-esteem. You might want to give them some of the words from page 39 to get them started.

❹ Allow approximately 15 minutes for this and then bring them back to the larger group.

❺ Invite the participants to read out their list of actions and write these on the large sheets of paper/flipchart.

ACTIVITY TWO

WHAT DO I DO TO MAKE PEOPLE FEEL GOOD OR BAD ABOUT THEMSELVES?

Discussion

High and low self-esteem can be strongly affected by how others treat us.

Have any of the participants felt that other people's actions have affected them by either raising or lowering their self-esteem?

Do they know of anyone who has been likewise affected?

Perhaps they can think of times when they may have affected someone's self-esteem through words or actions.

Variation

Once the participants have thought of actions that might affect someone's self-esteem, they could think of slogans that can remind us to think about how we talk or act towards others. This could then either be made into a poster or a t-shirt front. For example:

How would you feel if someone laughed at you?

ENDING POINTS

— If someone is having a bad day they might use words that hurt other people even though they don't mean to hurt them.

— Words and actions can have a very strong effect on how we feel about ourselves particularly if we hear the same words day after day. It is important to remember this when we are thinking about self-esteem.

— If someone is told that they are very clever all of the time they may begin to believe it; but likewise, if they are continually told that they are worthless, they may believe that too.

ACTIVITY TWO

WHAT DO I DO TO MAKE PEOPLE FEEL
GOOD OR BAD ABOUT THEMSELVES?

Examples of actions that can raise or lower self-esteem

Complimenting your mates or family

Gossiping about people

Ignoring others

Supporting a friend who needs help

Listening when your mate needs you to

Name-calling of someone who is different

Ganging up against someone

Laughing at other people

Spreading rumours about others

Making friends with someone who is lonely

ACTIVITY TWO

WHAT DOES IT FEEL LIKE TO HAVE A LOW SELF-ESTEEM?

Aim

To encourage participants to explore the different thoughts and feelings that individuals might experience when faced with low self-esteem.

You'll need

Large sheet of paper/flipchart
Felt-tip/marker pens
Pens
Photocopies of the problem letters (See pages 44-48)

Time

60 - 90 minutes

What to do

❶ Introduce the session by explaining to the group that they will be looking at the different feelings and thoughts of individuals when going through experiences which can affect self-esteem.

❷ Split the participants up into groups. Give each group one or two problem letters. Ask them to list the different kinds of thoughts and feelings that might be going on inside the individual who wrote the letters.

❸ Ideas might include - feeling insecure, anxious, distressed, unwanted, guilty, hurt, tired, unhappy, confused or unloved.

❹ Back in the larger group ask each group to read out their problem letter and the feelings they discussed.

❺ You could write out some of the ideas shared on a large sheet of paper/flipchart for everyone to see.

ACTIVITY THREE

WHAT DOES IT FEEL LIKE TO HAVE A LOW SELF-ESTEEM?

Discussion

You might want to pose a few questions for the participants to discuss, i.e.:

Do they think females and males have different levels of self-esteem?

Do they think self-esteem changes as you get older?

Do they think people from other cultures have different levels of self-esteem?

The aim of the discussion is to encourage participants to think about self-esteem from a number of different angles. It is not essential that you have concrete answers. It is essential however, to reinforce that people are all different regardless of their gender, age, culture and abilities. The way some of the above groups of people are slotted together, rather than seen as individuals, can affect self-esteem - for example, calling all old people 'wrinklies' can be very demeaning and offensive.

If you feel the group might want to learn at a more in-depth level about self-esteem this might be a good session to invite along somebody who has an understanding of the wider implications of self-esteem, such as a counsellor.

Variations

— Get groups to put their letters and replies on the wall and encourage others to walk around and read them.

— Use newspaper/magazine cuttings of different stories that highlight individuals who may have a low self-esteem, as relevant to young people, rather than the problem pages enclosed.

— Hire a video about good self-esteem and how to develop it. (See address lists on pages 74 and 75 for different organizations who may be able to help).

ACTIVITY THREE

WHAT DOES IT FEEL LIKE TO HAVE A LOW SELF-ESTEEM?

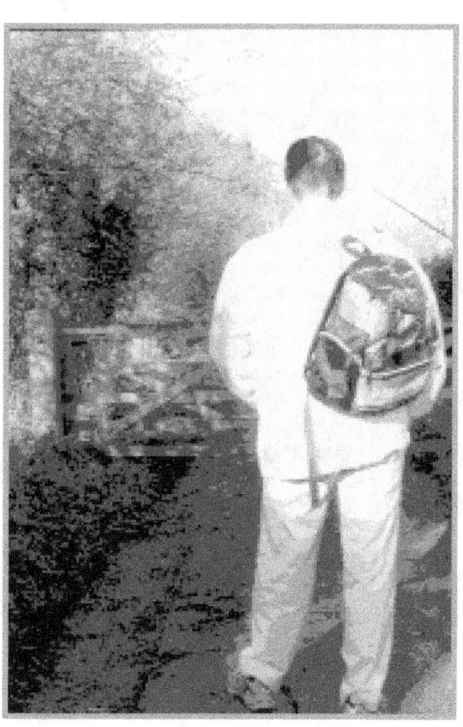

ENDING POINTS

— Emphasize the importance of:
   respecting cultural, gender and age differences in relation to self-esteem,
   understanding that fluctuating self-esteem is a normal part of life. One day you might feel great about yourself but then the next day something happens to make you feel down.

— Different people deal with self-esteem in different ways. What makes one person feel low may help to boost someone else.

ACTIVITY THREE

problem page

WHAT DOES IT FEEL LIKE TO HAVE A LOW SELF-ESTEEM?

Dear Sue,

I am a 13-year-old girl and I suffer really badly with spots. My mum took me to the doctor who gave me some cream but the spots are still there. I know they look really awful and I hate going to school in case any-one makes fun of me. A boy asked me out last week and I said no because I know I will get lots of spots and he will dump me. What can I do to make the spots go away?

From Tara, aged 13.

List the kind of thoughts and feelings that Tara might be having about her spots.

What could you do as her friend to help her feel better about herself?

_____

_____

_____

_____

_____

_____

_____

_____

_____

_____

_____

_____

_____

ACTIVITY THREE

WHAT DOES IT FEEL LIKE TO HAVE A LOW SELF-ESTEEM?

problem page

Dear Sue,

My dad left us when I was little and my brother and me live with our mum. She is a really great mum and I love her loads. The trouble is we don't have much money because she can only work when we are at school. All of my friends have designer clothes and expensive trainers but we have clothes from charity shops and from other people. I know it is not my mum's fault but I find it really hard when my friends go off on holiday to great places or come to school with computer games and things. There is a school trip coming up soon to France and I bet I will be the only one not going because we can't afford it. My friends don't make fun of me but I know they feel sorry for me.

Leroy aged 12.

List the kind of thoughts and feelings that Leroy might be experiencing about not having all of the things his friends have.
What could you do as his friend to help him feel better about himself?

_____
_____
_____
_____
_____
_____
_____
_____
_____
_____
_____
_____
_____
_____
_____

ACTIVITY THREE

problem page

WHAT DOES IT FEEL LIKE TO HAVE A LOW SELF-ESTEEM?

Dear Sue,
My family is very religious and so am I. The problem is that most of my friends at school are not religious at all and they can't understand why I am. My family gives part of their wages each month to the church and so we can't afford as many treats as my friends. I go to church on Sundays and we have prayer meetings during the week. I make friends really easily but when they find out about my reli-gion they go off and find other friends instead and I don't know what to do.
Mary aged 15.

List the kind of thoughts and feelings that Mary might be experiencing about her religion and her friends' reaction to it.
What could you do as her friend to help her feel better about herself?

ACTIVITY THREE

WHAT DOES IT FEEL LIKE TO HAVE A LOW SELF-ESTEEM?

Dear Sue,
At school one of the teachers keeps picking on me all the time. I don't know what I have done to make her hate me but she only ever picks on me and not my friends. If there is any trouble in the class I always get blamed for it even if I am sitting somewhere else. I am the only one who gets deten-tion from her and it is really upsetting me. I want to ask her what I have done wrong but I am scared that she will just shout at me. She has even told the headmaster that I am a troublemaker like my big brother was at school and he believed her. What can I do?
Gangan aged 15.

List the kind of thoughts and feelings that Gangan might be experiencing about the teacher's attitude towards her.
What could you do as her friend to help her feel better about herself?

ACTIVITY THREE

problem page

WHAT DOES IT FEEL LIKE TO HAVE A LOW SELF-ESTEEM?

Dear Sue,

Two months ago I lost my job at the local garage and that really knocked me. Since then I have run up quite a bit of debt as I have no income but I am smoking more and more. I left school with no qualifications so I don't think I will be able to get another job. My girlfriend keeps nagging me that we should get a place together and she told me last night that she thinks she is pregnant. I feel so desperate now, as I can't see my way out of this situation. The best thing for everyone would be if I killed myself. At least then I wouldn't have to try to sort out all these problems.

From Niall aged 17.

List the kind of thoughts and feelings that Niall might be experiencing because of the situation he finds himself in.

What could you do as his friend to help him feel better about himself?

_____
_____
_____
_____
_____
_____
_____
_____
_____
_____
_____
_____
_____
_____
_____

ACTIVITY THREE

WORD POWER

Aim

To help participants understand the effect of the power of words on someone's self-esteem.

You'll need

Photocopies of the role-play cards (see page 51)

Time

45 - 60 minutes

What to do

❶ Introduce the session by explaining that the group will be acting out some role-play to see how words can have an effect on someone's self-esteem.

❷ Split the participants up into groups and give each group a photocopy of one of the short role-play cards. Allow each group twenty minutes to read the cards, decide who is going to play which role and then rehearse the scenario.

❸ Back in the large group, give each group in turn the opportunity to do their role-play.

❹ When all the groups have done their role-play ask the following question:
Which of the role-plays would have helped a young person feel good about themselves and which would have made them feel bad about themselves?

❺ You might want to go through each scenario in turn or just have a general discussion.

ACTIVITY FOUR

WORD POWER

Discussion

Did the participants find it easy to play the roles in which they found themselves?

For those who were on the receiving end, how did it feel?

How did the others feel?

Which seemed to have more effect - the actions that would lower self-esteem or those that would build it?

Variation

— Rather than using the role-play cards provided, groups might like to make up their own situations.

— It is important to check that some of the role-plays are aimed at building self-esteem and some are aimed at undermining it.

ENDING POINTS

— We are all in a position to make people feel good or bad about themselves by what we say to them.

— Each young person needs to take responsibility for the part that they play in making others feel good or bad about themselves, regardless of whether the other person is younger, older or the same age.

ACTIVITY FOUR

WORD POWER

ROLE-PLAY CARDS

Situation 1 - Being bullied
(for 3 people)

You have just moved to a new area and started a new school where you don't know anyone. As you walk into the playground two other pupils come up to you and start taking the mickey out of some of your physical features, such as 'four eyes', 'fatso', 'stick insect',' titch', 'metal mouth' or 'big nose'.

Situation 2 - Being complimented
(for 4 people)

You have just had your belly-button pierced and you are not sure whether you like it or not. When you walk into your local café, three of your friends are there. When you show them your belly-button ring they start telling you how wonderful it is and how much it suits you.

Situation 3 - Making friends
(for 2 people)

You have just joined the local youth club where you don't know anyone. After sitting on your own for a while, one of the regulars comes over to your table. They ask if they can sit down and start talking to you, asking about yourself and telling you things about themselves. By the end of the evening you are firm friends.

Situation 4 - Spreading gossip
(for 3+ people)

When you walk into your classroom everyone stops talking and stares at you. After a little while they all start talking behind their hands while staring at you. When you ask what is going on they avoid answering. One person tells you that they have heard something really horrible about you and everyone is talking about it. You know it is not true but no one will listen to what you have to say.

Situation 5 - Listening
(for 3 people)

Life at home is getting very difficult. Your mum and dad keep rowing all the time and you are getting really worried that they are going to get a divorce. When you tell your friends about it, they listen to everything you are worried about and try to help and comfort you.

ACTIVITY FOUR

BULLYING & SELF-ESTEEM

Aim

To raise awareness about how bullying and being bullied can be linked to an individual's self-esteem.

You'll need

Photocopies of both the large and small 'bully/bullied' cards for each small group (see pages 55 and 56)

Time

45 - 60 minutes

What to do

❶ Introduce the session by explaining to the group that they will be exploring the effect of bullying on self-esteem.

❷ Split the participants up into smaller groups of 3 or 4. Give each group a set of the photocopied 'bully/bullied' cards. Ask them to place the 3 large cards face up on the table and place the smaller cards face down in a pile.

❸ Explain that each group member should pick a small card in turn and decide whether it goes on the BULLY, BULLIED or BOTH pile. Each card is then placed on whichever pile they think is correct.

❹ When all the cards have been selected and placed, the whole group should decide if they agree with where each card has been placed. If anyone thinks a card is wrong they can suggest reasons as to why they think it should be moved. It can then be moved if the group agrees.

❺ Back in the larger group ask where the groups had placed their cards and why.

ACTIVITY FIVE

BULLYING & SELF-ESTEEM

Discussion

Were some cards easy to place and some harder?

Which cards were placed on the BOTH pile and why?

Did the whole group place the same cards on the same piles? If not, invite explanations as to why they were different.

Variation

The words BULLY, BULLIED and BOTH can be written on large sheets of card or paper which are placed on the floor around the room.

One person reads out each of the smaller cards and the participants then choose which word they think fits that card.

They then walk to their chosen word and stand by it. If everyone does not agree invite a discussion as to why they think it should be different.

ENDING POINTS

— Self-esteem can be raised and lowered by all sorts of outside influences. Someone who is bullied may have very low self-esteem. That does not mean, however, that the bully has a high self-esteem. It is important for the group to understand that bullies may be hiding their own feelings of low self-worth and often need help just as much as the bullied.

— It is important to be sensitive to anyone in the group who may be being bullied or who may be a bully. Make sure that there is somewhere for them to go for help and advice if it is needed.

ACTIVITY FIVE

BULLYING & SELF-ESTEEM

BULLY

BULLIED

BOTH

ACTIVITY FIVE

BULLYING & SELF-ESTEEM

small bully/bullied cards

AFRAID	TEACHER	GENTLE
VAIN	PERSON WITH LEARNING DISABILITIES	LONER
AGGRESSIVE	PARENT	BOYFRIEND
SHY	LOW SELF-ESTEEM	GIRLFRIEND
DIFFERENT	GOOD SELF-ESTEEM	CHILD
UNATTRACTIVE	HURT	BROTHER OR SISTER
COWARD	SMALL	BOY
TIMID		GIRL

ACTIVITY FIVE

GET TO GRIPS WITH SELF-TALK!

Aim

To encourage the participants to recognize when they use negative self-talk and show them how to turn it around into positive self-talk.

You'll need

Large sheet of paper/flipchart
Small sheets of paper
Felt-tip/marker pens
Pens

Time

45 minutes

What to do

❶ Introduce the session by asking if any of the participants can tell the group what self-talk is.

❷ Make sure that all the participants understand that self-talk is how we talk to ourselves in our heads. It is like a running commentary on what is going on and what we think about it in order to make sense of the world. Self-talk might be something simple like reminding ourselves of the way to the shops or it could be something more negative like telling ourselves how useless we are.

❸ Explain that this session is going to explore negative self-talk and how to turn it into positive self-talk.

❹ Split the participants up into small groups and start off by giving them the examples of negative and positive self-talk (see page 59).

❺ Now ask each small group to write some more negative statements and turn them into positive statements.

❻ When everyone has several statements written, come back into the large group and invite them to read out their ideas. These can then be written on a large sheet of paper/flipchart and displayed where everyone can see them.

ACTIVITY SIX

GET TO GRIPS WITH SELF-TALK!

Discussion

Self-talk is important because most of us are talking silently to ourselves for much of the time. What we are saying can affect how we feel about ourselves and what we do. Negative self-talk can slowly wear away at our self-esteem until we believe everything we are saying to ourselves.

You might want to ask the participants if they are aware of this silent talking and what sort of things they think they say.

Encourage a discussion about the sort of things they might say and what affect this might have on their lives.

Variations

— Rather than using the negative self-talk statements provided, participants could write their own, together with how to turn them into positive statements.

— Participants could read out their answers in pairs with one giving the negative self-talk and the other giving the positive.

ENDING POINTS

— What we say to ourselves affects how we feel about ourselves.

— Everyone self-talks - it is normal, not a sign of madness. Most of the time we don't even notice we are doing it.

— The problem can arise if our self-talk is negative which in turn can make us feel lousy or can affect what we do.

— Instead of feeling miserable because someone has told you something horrible about yourself, turn it around and tell yourself that you are happy with yourself and that is all that matters.

ACTIVITY SIX

GET TO GRIPS WITH SELF-TALK!

Negative example:

"My dad says he thinks I am a no-hoper."

Positive example:

"I feel okay about myself and that is all that matters."

Negative example:

"I'm never going to get a girlfriend with these spots on my face."

Positive example:

"I'm a nice person with or without these spots."

examples of negative & positive self-talk

ACTIVITY SIX

AM I ASSERTIVE?

Aim

To help participants understand that they can be assertive without being aggressive.

You'll need

Felt-tip/marker pens
Pens
Photocopies of the assertiveness cards (see page 64)
Photocopies of the 10 assertiveness rules (see page 65)

Time

40 - 50 minutes

What to do

1 Introduce the session by explaining to the participants that people tend to deal with tricky situations using one of three ways:
— they might become aggressive by shouting or using physical strength;
— they might act passively by walking away or just agreeing with what is happening;
— or they can act assertively by ensuring that their opinion is heard but without resorting to aggression or passivity.
Usually, people with low self-esteem tend to be either aggressive or passive. Make sure that the participants understand what is meant by these behaviours and emphasize that the most productive behaviour is assertiveness. By acting out the situations in this activity they will learn how to be more assertive without being aggressive or passive.

2 Give each participant a photocopy of the 'assertiveness rules' (see page 65). Tell them that this is what they are aiming towards. Ask the participants to get into pairs and give each pair an 'assertiveness card' (see page 64). Allow them 10 minutes to run through their cards and decide who will do what and how.

3 Ask each pair in turn to act out the situations on their card. Remind them that they are not to become aggressive, no matter how unhelpful their partner is.

4 When all the situations have been acted out ask each pair to fill in their 'assertiveness rules' by ticking the boxes against the rules they feel they need to improve on, or against those they feel they act on already.

ACTIVITY SEVEN

AM I ASSERTIVE?

Discussion

Encourage a discussion on the advantages of using assertiveness and the disadvantages of using passivity and aggression.

Have they been in situations where they have used aggression or passivity and not had a favourable outcome? If they had been assertive would they have had a better result?

Variations

— Ask participants to make up their own situations in which they have to be assertive.

— Participants could all watch one particular TV soap or chat show and look out for signs of aggression, passivity or assertiveness.

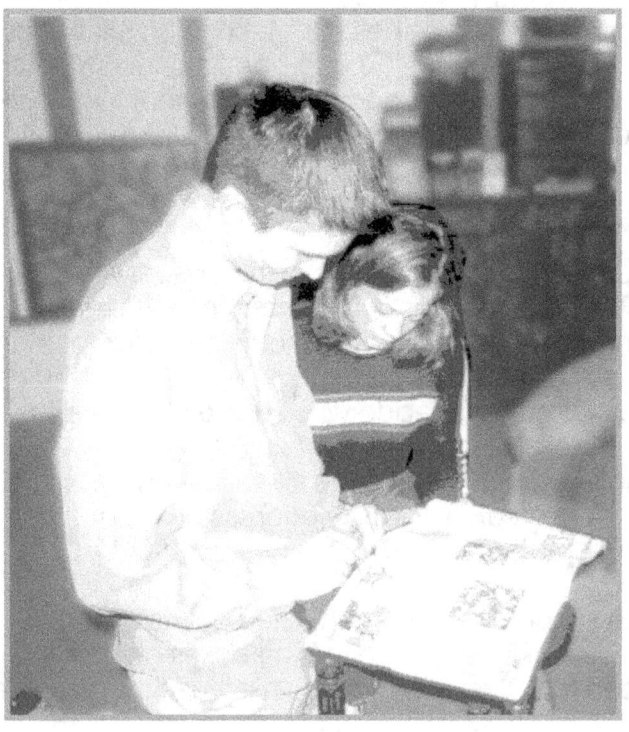

ACTIVITY SEVEN

AM I ASSERTIVE?

ENDING POINTS

Emphasize that assertiveness means:

— *respecting ourselves - who we are and what we do,*

— *taking responsibility for ourselves - how we feel and what we think and do,*

— *recognizing our own needs and wants,*

— *making it clear that other people understand what we feel and think,*

— *allowing ourselves to make mistakes,*

— *allowing ourselves to enjoy our successes,*

— *changing our minds if and when we choose,*

— *asking for time to think it over if we are not sure,*

— *asking for what we want rather than waiting for someone to offer,*

— *setting clear boundaries about what we will and will not do,*

— *recognizing that we have a responsibility towards others, not for others,*

— *respecting others and their right to be assertive too.*

ACTIVITY SEVEN

AM I ASSERTIVE?

assertiveness cards

1.
Tell your partner you are annoyed with him/her

2.
Pay your partner a genuine compliment.

3.
Ask your partner to return some money owing to you.

4.
Ask your partner not to smoke in your room.

5.
Tell your partner that you disagree with something he or she has said.

6.
Admit that you are wrong about something.

7.
Tell your partner about something you have done that you are very proud of.

8.
You have to meet your partner to exchange some important papers. Arrange to meet him or her at a specific time and in a specific place. Make sure your partner agrees to turn up.

ACTIVITY SEVEN

AM I ASSERTIVE?

In becoming more assertive a person develops an awareness of not only what they say but also how they say it.

	I need to improve on	I already do
1. First decide what you want. This is important as otherwise everyone will be confused, including you.	☐	☐
2. Say what you want clearly and be specific. "I'll meet you at 2 pm by the post office", rather than "I'll see you in town sometime tomorrow afternoon".	☐	☐
3. Emphasize what you say by how you say it. If something is serious - look serious. If you are laughing when you say something serious the other person often doesn't know what to believe.	☐	☐
4. Don't let yourself get side-tracked. Say what you want and if necessary repeat yourself. Don't allow the other person to change the subject or bully you into changing your mind.	☐	☐
5. Listen to the other person. Like you, they have the right to their own opinion.	☐	☐
6. Aim for a win-win situation. Being assertive isn't about getting your own way all the time. A compromise that works equally well for both parties is much better.	☐	☐
7. Keep good eye contact. If you can look directly at the other person it conveys honesty and assertion. Looking away signifies passivity.	☐	☐
8. Good upright posture also shows assertiveness. Standing or sitting slouched or huddled up does not convey good self-esteem or assertiveness.	☐	☐
9. Don't turn statements into questions by adding "don't you think?" on the end. This shows that you are unsure and seeking reassurance. If it is your opinion, own it and tell them "I think...".	☐	☐
10. Think about the words you use. 'I can't', 'I have to', and 'I imagine' are all passive words. Use 'I won't', 'I choose to' and 'I know' instead. These are much more assertive words and show that you have good self-esteem.	☐	☐

ACTIVITY SEVEN

AGREEING THE GROUND RULES!

Aim

To get participants thinking about what kind of support they would like from the others in their group.

You'll need

Small sheets of paper
Felt-tip/marker pens
Pens
Tape recorder for Rap

Time

45 - 60 minutes

What to do

❶ Introduce the session by explaining to the group that it is very easy not to realize that you are knocking someone and lowering their self-esteem.

❷ Their task in this session is to design a **SET OF RULES** for the whole group to agree on.
It is to be a guide to how not to lower self-esteem and how to help build it. Examples might include:

'If you can't say something nice, don't say anything'
'If someone does something well, tell them'

❸ Split the participants into small groups and ask them to discuss ideas for their **SET OF RULES**

❹ They will then need to plan how they are going to introduce their ideas to the rest of the group. For example:

Plan a small role play and act it out, to highlight the points they want to make,
design a leaflet,
write a rap and then perform it,
write a list and get everyone to sign it.

❺ Give each small group the opportunity to do their presentations and encourage questions and discussion.

ACTIVITY EIGHT

AGREEING THE GROUND RULES!

Discussion

You may want to broaden the discussion by asking participants whether they had any thoughts about how they could communicate a collective set of ground rules to others in their organization and what user-friendly name they could give to them.

Variation

If you want to make this activity shorter you could have a large group discussion about how young people want to be respected and supported by others and then do just one set of rules.

SET OF RULES

ENDING POINTS

— Emphasize the importance of being allowed to make mistakes without being criticised and to be told you have done well when a task has been completed.

— Everyone is entitled to respect from their class mates, friends, teachers, boss and/or work colleagues.

ACTIVITY EIGHT

Mind Matters

WHERE DO WE GO FOR HELP?

Aim

To raise awareness about national and local organizations which are available to help young people.

You'll need

Small sheets of paper
Felt-tip/marker pens
Pens
Photocopies of the quiz (see page 73)
List of names and address of local and national support systems,, (pages 74 and 75), directories, helpline numbers, phone books and leaflets that link to the quiz scenarios on page 73.

Time

60 - 90 minutes

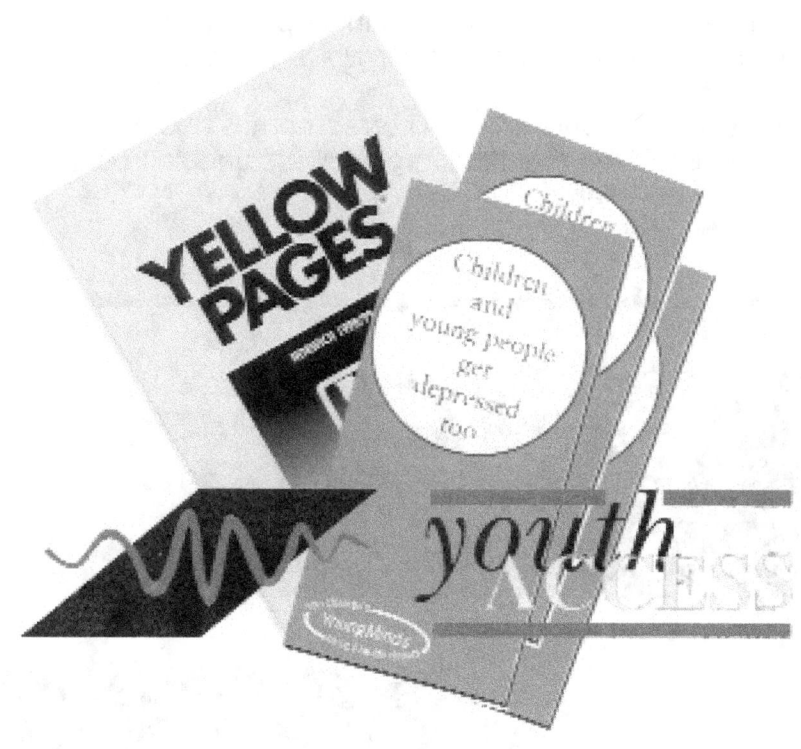

ACTIVITY NINE

What to do

❶ Explain to the group that there are all sorts of helplines, support groups and organizations which support people who are faced with problems. By filling in the quiz (see page 73) participants will explore many of these resources for people in different situations.

❷ Split the participants into fours and ask them to read through the quiz. Using the list of names and addresses or leaflets they should find at least one organization for each scenario.

❸ Bring the group back together and invite participants to share which organizations they picked for which scenario.

It is important that you have the correct names and addresses for each scenario in the event that groups were unable to answer some of the questions.

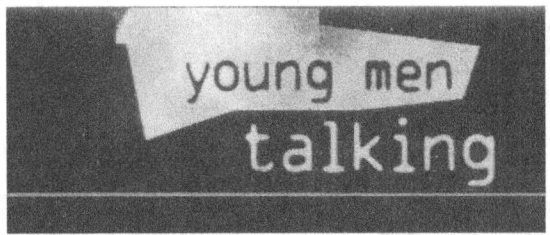

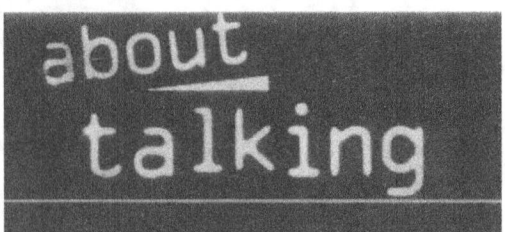

ACTIVITY NINE

WHERE DO WE GO FOR HELP?

Discussion

Did the participants pick the same organizations for each scenario? If not, invite the participants to explain why they chose the particular organization.

Encourage a discussion about the kinds of concerns that would encourage and/or hinder them when approaching a helping service if they were in need of help.

How might they be able to overcome some of the concerns in order to obtain the help that they require? For example:

Concern	_Solution_
Scared to go alone	take a friend
Not knowing what to say	write down beforehand important points you want to make

Variations

— Using the list of names and addresses and leaflets etc. the participants could design a poster or web page to advertize the help that is available to young people.

— You could arrange to have somebody from a local support organization to come and talk about the work of their organization and how it supports young people.

— Using the Internet to find helping services (if the equipment is available,) may provide additional information that is not in the leaflets and posters you have obtained.

ACTIVITY NINE

WHERE DO WE GO FOR HELP?

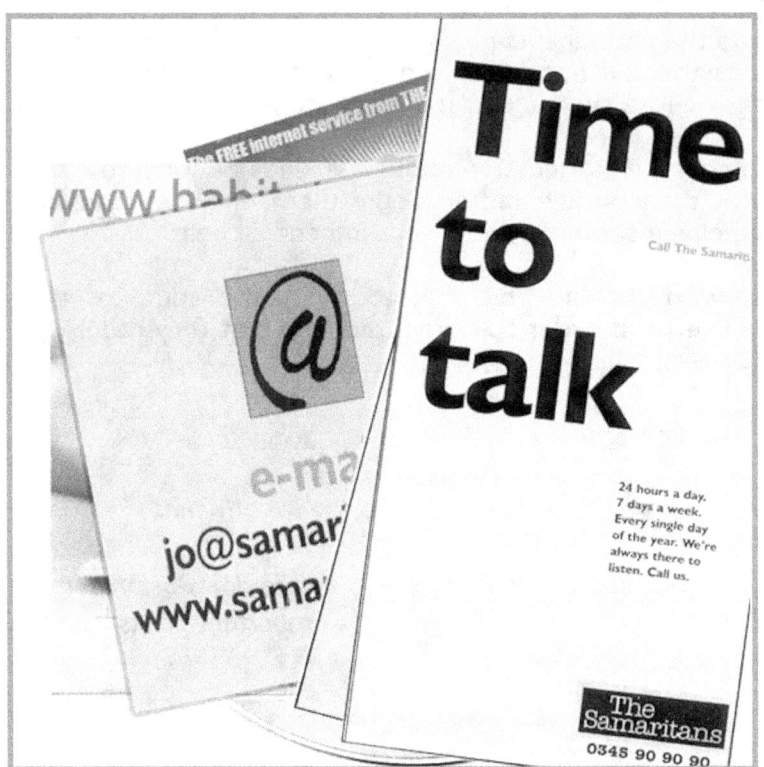

ENDING POINTS

— Many young people do support their friends and family when they are feeling unhappy, rejected or worried and that is important.

— Sometimes, however, a young person may need help from an agency or professional.

— The way you respond to a mate who is seeking professional help might influence their willingness to accept it or not.

— For example, if you laugh at them for getting professional help they are going to have difficulty in feeling supported by others.

ACTIVITY NINE

WHERE DO WE GO FOR HELP?

QUIZ

1. One of your friends has been smoking for a little while and has decided they want to give up but they are finding it really difficult. Where could they go for help?

2. A friend has told you that she thinks she might be pregnant. She doesn't want to tell her mum or anyone at school but she's scared. She needs practical help. Where could she go for this help?

3. A friend has told you that he is really unhappy at home. He feels no one in his family loves him and he is planning to run away from home. Where could he go for help?

4. One of your friends lives in care and is unhappy where she is. She has spoken to her social worker but he did not really listen. Where could she go for help?

5. Your friend has asthma. He is seeing a doctor but his symptoms are really bad and it is getting to him. Where could he go for help and advice?

6. Your friend's mum has left home and he is finding it really difficult living with his dad who is still upset and depressed. You have listened to all your friend's worries but he still needs more help. Where could he go for this help?

7. You have noticed that some older boys are bullying one of your friends at school. His clothes are always torn and they take his dinner money. He has spoken to the teacher but it is still happening. Where could he go for help and advice?

8. Your friend has been through a lot of family trouble just lately. She has told you that she can't cope anymore and you are worried that she is thinking of attempting suicide. Where could she go for help and advice?

9. Your friend left school last year and since then hasn't found a job. He has no money and he has told you he is really depressed. Where could he go for help?

10. A girl the same age as you has just moved into your street. She is from a different culture to the rest of the people in your street and she is finding it very hard to fit in and make new friends. Is there somewhere in the area that she could ask for help and support?

ACTIVITY NINE

WHERE DO WE GO FOR HELP?

Helpful Addresses

Alcoholics Anonymous
Tel: 020 7352 3001

Careline
Tel: 020 8514 1177
A confidential telephone counselling service for people of any age with any problem.

Childline
FREEPOST 1111 London N1 0BR
Free 24 hour helpline 0800 1111

CRUSE
Cruse House, 126 Sheen Road, Richmond,
Surrey, TW9 1UR
Tel: 020 8940 4818
Offers help to anyone who has suffered the loss of a friend or relative.

Eating Disorders Association
National helpline 01603 621414
Youth helpline 01603 765050

Gamblers Anonymous
Tel: 020 7384 3040

Health Information Service
Tel: 0800 66 55 44
Provides information to the general public about health-related issues.

London Lesbian and Gay helpline
Tel: 020 7837 7324
For anyone who needs support regarding their sexuality.

Mental Health Programme
Health Education Authority, Trevelyn House,
30 Great Peter Street, London SW1P 2HW
Tel: 020 7413 2009
Provides information and resources for World Mental Health Day campaign.

ACTIVITY NINE

WHERE DO WE GO FOR HELP?

Helpful Addresses (cont.)

Message Home
Tel: 0500 700 740
A confidential helpline for those who have left home
or have run away to send a message home and/or get
help and advice.

National Council for One Parent Families
255 Kentish Town Road, London NW5
Tel: 020 7428 5400 Freephone 0800 0185026
Provides information and advice for lone parents.

The Relaxation for Living Trust
168-170 Oatlands Drive, Weybridge, Surrey KT13 9ET
Tel: 01932 831000

Sexwise
Freephone 0800 282930
Provides information, advice and guidance for young
people on issues including sexuality contraception, safe
sex, feelings, emotions and relationships.

The Samaritans
24 hour helpline: 0345 90 90 90

Young Minds
102-108 Clerkenwell Road, London EC1M 5SA
Tel: 020 7336 8445
www.youngminds.org.uk

Young People's Health Network
c/o Sally Taylorson, Health Education Authority,
Trevelyn House, 30 Great Peter Street,
London SW1P 2HW
Tel: 020 7413 2630
For information, advice, and the sharing of good prac-
tice for workers working alongside young people on
health issues.
www.hea.org.uk/yphn/index.html

Youth Access
1a Taylors Yard, 97 Alderbrook Road,
London SW12 8AD
Tel: 020 8772 9900
Will put you in touch with local contacts for
counselling, advice and information.

All details correct at time of going to press

ACTIVITY NINE

WHAT DO YOU KNOW NOW?

Aim

To enable the participants to understand how much they have learnt by using a fun activity to finish with.

You'll need

Pens
Photocopies of the human bingo cards (one per person) on page 79

Time
45 minutes

What to do

❶ Hand out the copies of the human bingo cards.

❷ Allow 15 - 20 minutes for the participants to go around the room asking each other questions and filling in the relative bingo card boxes.

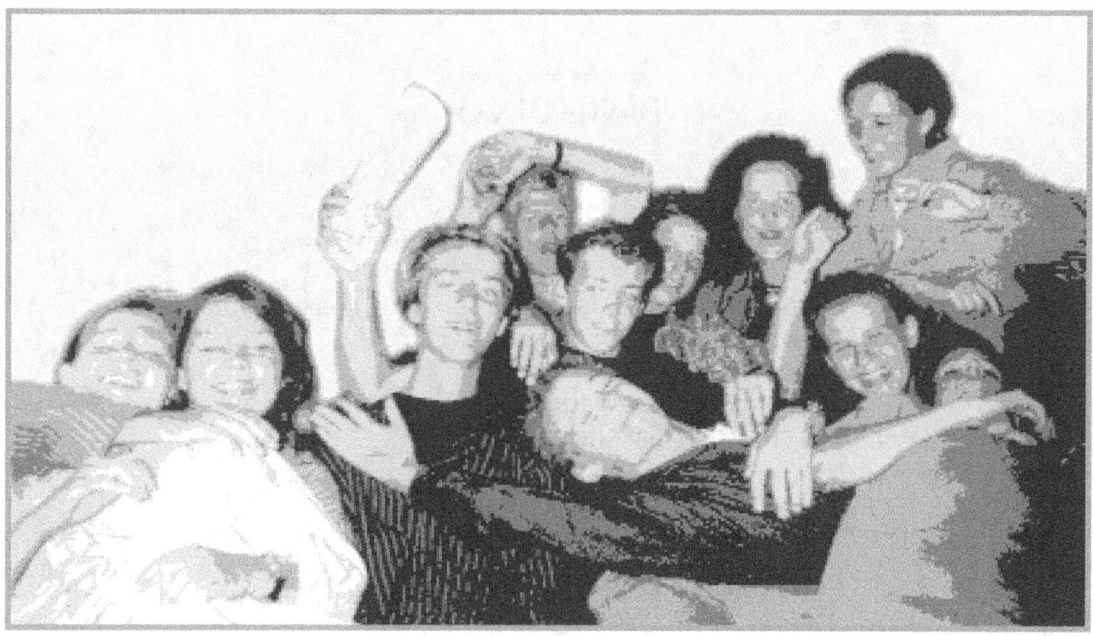

ACTIVITY TEN

WHAT DO YOU KNOW NOW?

Discussion

When you bring the group back together go through each question and allow people to call out an answer if they wish.

Acknowledge all correct answers but sensitively clarify any wrong answers.

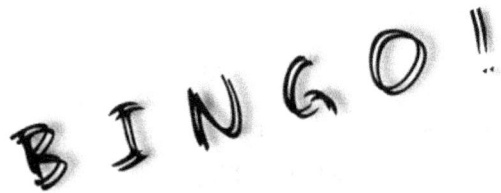

ENDING POINTS

— The last questions in the bingo card game will enable you to end the programme in a lively way.

— It is important to thank people for their ideas about future learning in relation to self-esteem.

— Tell people you will be around to answer any questions they may have.

ACTIVITY TEN

WHAT DO YOU KNOW NOW?

Find someone who can think of three different positive phrases associated with self-esteem. 1. 2. 3. Signed	Find someone who can name three different ways to be assertive. 1. 2. 3. Signed ....
Shake hands with someone and ask if they have enjoyed learning about self-esteem. Signed	Find someone who can think of two things they will miss about not being in the group anymore. 1. 2. Signed ....
Find someone who can tell you the two ways they best learn about self-esteem e.g. reading, listening, playing games. 1. 2. Signed	Find someone who can identify one more thing they would like to learn about self-esteem. Signed ....
Find someone who can tell you two ways of helping someone who is suffering low self-esteem. 1. 2. Signed	Find someone who can tell you three places to go for help with self-esteem matters. 1. 2. 3. Signed ....

ACTIVITY TEN

Project
Part four

Young Men Talking about Talking

"Young men are often viewed as difficult, uncommunicative and unwilling to reveal their thoughts and emotions. Being helped to value and extend their ability to communicate with each other, and other adults, is central to their finding positive solutions in a rapidly changing world."

During the past three years Youth Clubs UK has supported a number of youth organizations to develop young men's projects. Using four groundbreaking projects in Liverpool, Cheshire, Cornwall and Leicester a video was produced describing projects that addressed young men's issues. It includes footage of workers undertaking a range of activities with young men and how they used different approaches to encourage communication. Outlined below is a description of how one of those projects evolved from an initial pilot project.

The Young Men's Project Cheshire Phase Two

The history

Following phase one of the Young Men's project, I had kept in touch with most of the group through their local youth centre. Many of the young men had been involved in various projects and activities including:

— Drama and performance
— Community initiatives
— Youth Achievement Awards
— Running a junior youth club

It was decided to continue working with the same group for phase two of the project for a number of reasons:

— the group were keen to do more,
— the young men had developed significantly and we were keen to see them move on further,
— we were the only one of the pilot projects still working with the same group and wanted to look at the benefits of working with one group for a sustained period of time.

The group

Inevitably, because of the time involved, there had been some changes to the group. Some of the young men had moved away, lost touch or simply decided not to become involved. We were left with five of the original group plus one new member who had become involved in many of the interim activities mentioned.

Phase two

The structure for the project involved three aspects:

1. Social activity days
2. Discussion work
3. Residential

Social Activity Days:

There were four days which were chosen in consultation between the workers and the young men, taking into account that we wanted the group to gain a range of new experiences and that we had a budget to work to. The days chosen were:

1. Day at Manchester Science Museum
2. Evening theatre trip to Blackpool
3. Outdoor day at the Crocky Trail
4. High level ropes course at the Conwy Centre

The young men behaved impeccably during each visit and were enthusiastic about all of the activities. Many had been to the Science museum as children, but were now more interested in how things worked and made sure they saw every section of the museum. The visit to the theatre was not ideal; as none of the group had ever been to a theatre before, we were keen to share this experience, however, because of the time of year, the only choice available was 'Summer Holiday'. Despite being incredibly corny, the group mostly enjoyed the performance and did experience live theatre! Day three was chosen as a budget day out because the group were so eager about day four, despite the expense. This fourth day was chosen as the favourite for all members of the group and provided a chance for the development of teamwork, confidence, support and encouragement and communication skills.

Discussion work:

The group work undertaken in phase one was seen as an important step in encouraging the young men to share ideas, opinions and thoughts. Experience of the working methods of the group meant that I could anticipate, to some extent, which activities they would respond to. Topics chosen in consultation with the group were:

— offending and the influence of friends
— anger and self control
— mental health and stress
— prejudice

Role-play was a major part of each session as this had proved to be a successful way for the young men to share their feelings and explore their attitudes. Other groupwork methods used were:

— brainstorm
— card exercises
— photopack
— use of magazine/newspaper articles
— mime
— agree/disagree exercises
— general discussion

The residential:

To finish off the project, we went on a three-day residential to the Pioneer Centre in Kidderminster. The idea for this residential had developed from wanting to move one step further with the group, but realising that they were not yet ready to go into other youth groups with a peer education project. Other factors were the enthusiasm of the group for role-play and how much they had enjoyed participating in the Youth Clubs UK video.

The residential was designed to produce a fly-on-the-wall type video, showing the processes involved in working with a group of young men towards a performance. A local video company was hired to document the weekend and they filmed the process at each step. Before the residential, the young men had chosen drugs misuse, prejudice and sexual health as the three issues which they perceived to be of most relevance to young men of their age. These provided our starting point.

Throughout the weekend we ran a series of workshops in order to develop the play. We worked on:

— warm ups
— plot development
— character development
— scene development
— prop and costume making
— rehearsal
— performance

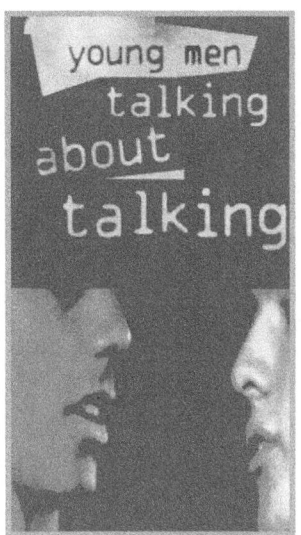

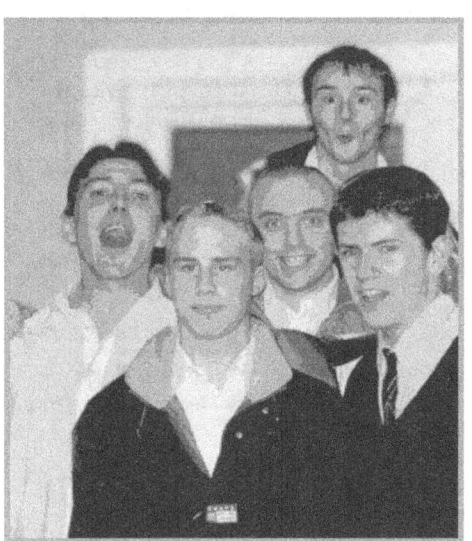

We also had a trip to a local bowling alley on the second night of the residential. This broke up the 'work' and gave the young men an opportunity to let off steam in an informal environment.

The young men developed many skills over the weekend, such as negotiation, creativity, teamwork, and co-operation. They also produced a play consisting of 12 short scenes which examined young people's use of illegal drugs, gangs and exclusion amongst young people and the effects of family stress. Extracts from each workshop along with individual interviews with the young men, footage of other aspects of the weekend and the final performance, were collated into a video which is to be available to workers wanting to undertake similar work with young men.

Important learning

There were a number of factors which were significant in working with this group of young men:

In discussion work:

— The activity stimulus used was important. The group responded best to a variety of short activities and would lose concentration if one activity went on for too long.

— Long negotiated breaks were scheduled. This enabled the young men to play physical games and use up some of their energy. It also provided a time when informal conversations could develop and ideas could be explored or developed outside of the 'formal' session.

— An established structure was important. Each session followed a similar structure, beginning with a warm up, followed by one or two short activities, a break in the middle, a role-play exercise with performance and ending with a simple evaluation.

— The space used. It was important that we had the building to ourselves and were able to use a small enclosed room with comfy chairs.

In activity work:

— Interspersing the groupwork with exciting and/or physical activity helped to maintain the momentum of the project.

— Encouraging the group to choose the activity days themselves meant that they were committed to the choices, but discussing these choices with them ensured a variety of experiences.

— Taking the group away from Ellesmere Port for each activity day meant that more value was placed on the visits and they were less likely to abuse this privilege.

During the residential:

— The young men were given options from which to develop the structure for their performance. This helped them to devise the piece quickly, but ensured that the idea was still their own.

— Using the medium of role-play and character development meant that the young men could discuss the issues in some depth whilst remaining at a safe distance from their feelings.

—Things such as prop and costume making and the bowling trip meant that the format of the weekend stayed varied and the group maintained their concentration.

Young People's Evaluation

Young people were asked to fill in evaluation forms of the project. Quoted below are some of the points made.

Discussion workshops

"It showed me how far I was willing to go, that was interesting to look at."

"(I enjoyed the session on) prejudice because it is one of the main problems in society."

"The discussion on ageism (was the most important to me) because it has affected me the most."

"I was able to tell people what I thought."

Activity days

"The museum was great and I really enjoyed it."

"The Opera House was enjoyable and I thought the show was very good. There wasn't anything I didn't enjoy about the trip."

"I thought the Crocky trail was brill, it was fun and a laugh, I fell in a lot and got dirty."

"The day at the Conwy Centre was the best thing I have done ever in my life, no words really describe it, it was amazing."

"I enjoyed the ropes course because at first I was scared but everyone helped me and now I have more confidence."

Residential

"I liked the fact that we could make our own characters and our own play and were not told what to do and who to be, it let us develop our own ideas."

"Everyone worked together and I didn't feel excluded from the groups.

"The warm up games were fun and the practising for the performance was challenging because we had to remember our lines."

Overall evaluation

Knowing the group so well was a definite advantage in phase two of the project. The production of the video was fairly costly and I needed to be sure that the group would work throughout the weekend, which they did. I also knew which activities they would respond to and how to structure the weekend in order for it to be successful.

Having two residentials at a 12-month interval demonstrated how much the young men had developed over the course of the project. Social skills such as listening, co-operation, negotiation and communication had progressed in leaps and bounds.

Throughout the residential itself, it was rewarding to watch the self-esteem and confidence of some members increase over the three days. The quietest member of the group took on the main part of the play and blossomed in the role, he was able to be the centre of attention during rehearsal and his confidence on return from the residential had also increased. The intense nature of the weekend meant that the young men did have to work hard, but the presence of the video camera helped to focus them, they also enjoyed the attention of the camera, they seemed to feel valued and their self-esteem was boosted.

The Young Men's project has, in my opinion, been a huge success. Although it has been a slow process, this seemed to work well with the young men as it took time to build up their confidence and security within the project. Having phase two as a development, rather than a continuation of phase one, ensured that the group and the project moved on. As well as being a success for those young men involved, we have also produced a resource which will, hopefully, be informative to those workers wanting to pursue work with young men.

Sam Dutton
Youth Worker
Cheshire & Wirral Federation of Youth Clubs

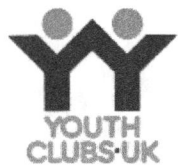

YOUTH
CLUBS·UK

Additional useful resources from Youth Clubs U.K.

Other titles in the Mind Matters series
> **Loss & Grief** - 'It hurts'
> **Stress** - 'Life's hassles'
> **Actions** - 'Should I - shouldn't I?'
> **Relationships** - 'Work it out!'

Video   Young Men Talking About Talking

For: Youth workers, Health workers, Managers.
Key themes: Young Men, Mental Health, Emotions, Communication.

This valuable video is for youth workers, teachers, social workers and anyone wishing to engage in positive communication with young men.

Using four groundbreaking projects in innercity Liverpool, Cheshire, Cornwall and Leicester, this video suggests ways in which you can start encouraging young men to talk about their lives, feelings, attitudes and behaviour. It includes footage of workers undertaking a range of activities with young men, also of workers describing different approaches to their work and how they utilise those approaches to encourage communication.

Manual   You Can't be Serious - Mental Health Activities for Peer Educators

For: Peer Educators

Peer education is one of the most effective ways of getting across a health message to young people. 'You Can't be Serious' contains guidance on the role of a peer educator, background information on mental health issues, activities for use by peer educators and a case study. Themes covered include: bullying, understanding mental health, feelings, loss and grief, friendship and sources of help.

By Marilyn Harvey

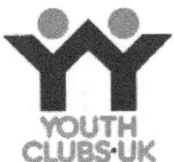

Manual   A Framework for Peer Learning

For: Peer Educators

Identifies the key practical problems and dilemmas that workers are likely to meet in setting up a peer education programme. It presents guidelines for action, outlines for recruitment and training, plans for follow up reviews and activity sheets.

By Marilyn Harvey

Manual   Yes Me

For: Peer Educators

A self-development programme for peer educators. This will guide young people through a process which will develop their understanding and teach the skills required to facilitate a peer learning group.

By Marilyn Harvey and Gillian Smith

Booklet   Analysis of a 'healthy' Health Allliance

This booklet offers an analysis of a Youth Clubs UK programme that uses the co-operative aproach to health education currently urged by the government. It shows how youth workers have much to offer to other agencies which are trying to reach young people.

By Alan Rogers

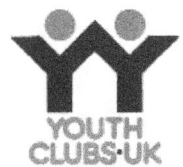

Posters   Talking About Ourselves

A set of 3 full colour A2 posters which feature strong, positive visual images and words of young white women. They act as a useful discussion starter and as an aid to combating sexism and discrimination. Bold statements say "Give me my space", "Never judge me" and "What sort of girl are you? - A Builder".

Produced by young white women in Sussex with support from Jane Fox

All available from:

Youth Clubs UK,
   20/24 Kirby Street, London EC1N 8TS
   Telephone 020 7242 4045
   Fax 020 7242 4125
   Registered Charity Number 306066
   VAT number 232464187

   Please allow 28 days for delivery

The latest catalogue on Youth Clubs UK's full current range of resource material is available by contacting Youth Clubs UK at the above address.